I0420665

Ultimate Apple Cider Vinegar For Weight Loss Guide!

Apple Cider Vinegar For Weight Loss

How To Lose Weight Fast And Increase Health With 101 Delicious Apple Cider Vinegar Meal Recipes Under 30 Minutes!

Sarah Brooks

STOP!!! Before you read any further....Would you like to know the Secrets of Body Transformation?

If your answer is yes, then you are not alone. Thousands of people are looking for the secret to rapidly burn body fat, keep the weight off, become healthier, and truly transform their body and life for good.

If you have been searching for these answers without much luck, you are in the right place!

Not only will you gain incredible insight in this book, but because I want to make sure to give you as much value as possible, right now for a limited time you can get full **100% FREE access to a VIP bonus EBook** entitled **THE 7 KEYS TO BODY TRANSFORMATION!**

Just Go Here For Free Instant Access:

www.liveFitVIP.com

Legal Notice

Disclaimer Notice

Table Of Contents

Introduction

I want to thank you and congratulate you for purchasing the book, "Apple Cider Vinegar For Weight Loss".

This "Apple Cider Vinegar for Weight Loss" book contains proven steps and strategies on how to use apple cider vinegar for various recipes.

Apple cider vinegar is one of the natural products that have many benefits. The vinegar is made from fermented apples. It is a strong anti-inflammatory and antibacterial agent that can cleanse the body from toxins and impurities. It can also help you lose weight gradually if you add it regularly to your recipes.

You can also use it to create your own tonic and drink. This book contains information on how you can detox and lose weight using apple cider vinegar. The last chapter discuses the other uses of apple cider vinegar from home use to beauty and medicinal use.

Thanks again for purchasing this book, I hope you enjoy it!

Chapter 1: Introduction To Apple Cider Vinegar

Apple cider vinegar is made from fermented apples. Apple cider vinegar has been used for several centuries for its medicinal and therapeutic benefits.

Apple cider vinegar vs. Distilled vinegar

Vinegar is commonly found in any household kitchen. It is a very versatile and can be used in various meal recipes. Holistic practitioners also believe that it can remove toxins in the body effectively without using chemicals. Distilled and apple cider vinegar are vinegars that are made in different ways.

Vinegar is a solution made from acetic acid. The strength of the vinegar depends on the amount of acid in it. Acetic acid is different from diluted acid. It is stable enough to be stored at room temperature because the acids serve as natural preservative.

The process of making vinegar is quite simple. It involves natural sugars from vegetables and fruits and fermentation to make vinegar. The process usually has two stages: alcoholic and acid fermentation.

In the first stage of fermentation, the yeast breaks down the starch and transforms it into an alcohol. The second stage involves microorganisms that ferment the alcohol and turn it into acetic acid.

Apple cider vinegar has been the preferred vinegar in America where apples were abundant. It was initially used to preserve foods before refrigerators were invented. Distilled vinegar on the other hand is made from distilled alcohol that goes through the second stage of fermentation. It can be made from any products that contain starch such as potatoes, rice and barley. Distilled vinegar contains less acid than apple cider vinegar.

Both vinegars can be used the same way but people typically use apple cider vinegar more because it has a lighter taste compared to distilled vinegar. Diluted vinegar also has practical household uses because of its disinfectant and cleansing properties.

Chapter 2: How To Use Apple Cider For Weight Loss

There are many fad diets in the market that promises great weight loss effects. Apple cider vinegar has been said to aid gradual weight loss. It can be easy to get attracted to products that promises fast weight loss but studies show that these have short term effect. If your body loses weight too quickly, your body mechanism will adjust so that you gain the weight back just as easily.

How does it work?

There is a Japanese study that shows that obese people who took 30 ml of apple cider vinegar everyday experienced fewer cravings and had lower blood sugar level after meals. There is enough medical evidence that shows that lower insulin levels can encourage weight loss.

The most common explanation is organic enzymes and acid in the apple cider vinegar that can successfully reduce your appetite. The study also showed that apple cider vinegar can speed up your metabolism even at rest so you burn more calories throughout the day.

How long should you take apple cider vinegar?

Apple cider vinegar can help you lose weight slowly. Studies show that gradual weight loss is healthier for the body.

Each person has a unique metabolism and lifestyle habits. It can be difficult to gauge for certain just how much weight you are going to lose. Some people lose weight just after one month while it might take a slightly longer time for other people.

How can you speed up your weight loss?

Nothing can still beat a healthy lifestyle when it comes to weight loss. A healthy diet rich in whole foods, regular exercise, stress management and toxin avoidance can greatly help you reach your ideal weight.

Increase the length of time or intensity of your exercise. Doctor recommends 30 minutes of moderate physical activity 3-4 times in a week. However, if you want to lose weight, you will have to do more than that. Aim for 40 minutes five days in a week and gradually increase your intensity when you become comfortable. Exercising regularly can help increase your metabolism.

Reduce your sugar consumption and avoid refined sugar as much as possible. Food products rich in sugar are rich in empty calories which do not provide your body with the necessary nutrients to function. Opt for natural sweeteners such as fruits, honey or maple syrup instead.

Chapter 3: Using Apple Cider Vinegar To Detox Your Body

Many people praise the medicinal benefits of apple cider vinegar. Apple cider vinegar is a very versatile product that can be used in recipes and beauty treatments.

The need for detox

The human body has its own system of detoxification. However, people are exposed to many toxins from environmental pollutants to free radicals from foods. You can help your body by using natural products like apple cider vinegar and speed up the detoxification process.

The detox properties of ACV

Apple cider vinegar is rich in minerals and nutrients that can cleanse the body of toxins. It also contains enzymes that can prevent the accumulation of waste in the body before it causes damage. It can also help improve digestion and aid in bowel movement.

In eastern medicine, apple cider vinegar is also used to improve the circulation of lymph in the body. It helps to detoxify the liver and purify the blood. The enzymes in the vinegar also break down the bad cholesterol in the blood and prevent it from clogging your arteries.

Apple cider vinegar can help maintain the right pH level in the body and protect it from inflammation. Lastly, apple cider vinegar can cleanse the lymph nodes and improve the body's immune system.

What type of apple cider vinegar to use?

The type of apple cider that you choose to use can affect its potency. Pure apple cider vinegar is the best option. It is made from organic apples that have been fermented to make vinegar. You should always choose unfiltered and unprocessed apple cider vinegar. It should have the "mother", the cloudy matter that either floats or sinks in the bottle. The mother is rich in trace minerals and enzymes that boost the benefits of the apple cider vinegar. Always shake the bottle before you use it.

How to use apple cider for detox?

You can use apple cider vinegar in several ways:

- Internal Use

You should always remember that apple cider vinegar is very acidic so you should not drink it pure because it can burn your throat and destroy your teeth. Although apple cider vinegar is acidic in nature, it has an alkaline effect once consumed.

The simplest way to consume apple cider is to dilute 2 tablespoon of vinegar with one glass of water and consume it before meals. You can also add it to your recipes and drinks.

If you plan to use apple cider vinegar long term, make sure that you consult your doctor first because it may interact with other medications for diabetes and heart disease.

- Apple Cider Vinegar Bath

The skin is the largest organ in the body. It is has a major role in keeping the body clean. You can jumpstart the detoxification process by having a detoxifying bath.

The smell of vinegar may make you uncomfortable but there are benefits in using apple cider vinegar on the skin. Add one cup of apple cider vinegar and one cup of Epsom salt into your warm bath water. Soak for 20 minutes then rinse with water. The apple cider vinegar can make your skin become smooth and supple. It is also effective in curing skin irritations and bacterial infections.

- Facial Wash

One of the most effective and economical way to get rid of acne is by using apple cider vinegar toner. It has strong antibacterial and anti-inflammatory properties that can help reduce acne. Just be sure to dilute the vinegar in water before using it. Avoid sensitive areas of the face like the nose and eyes.

Chapter 4: Making Your Own Organic Apple Cider Vinegar

Just like apple juice, the best apple cider vinegar is made from fresh and organic apples. Some people may not have a steady supply of apple cider vinegar so making your own batch can be convenient. You will also save more money in making your own apple cider vinegar especially if you tend to use it a lot on recipes and food.

Apple Cider Vinegar from Scraps

You can make vinegar from the peels and cores of apples. This method only takes about 1-2 months to complete.

Peel and core of apples
1 liter of water
3 tbsp honey

Procedure:

1. Wash the apples. Cut the core and peel.
2. Air dry it until it turns brown. Place the core and peel in a large jar. Fill the jar with water.
3. Cover the jar with cheesecloth then secure with rubber band.
4. Store it in a cool and dry place. Make sure that you stir it every day. You can use notes to help you remember to stir the mixture.
5. Strain the mixture and remove the scraps. Taste the vinegar and adjust the taste as necessary.
6. Transfer into a clean bottle. Remember to shake before you use.

Apple Cider Vinegar from Whole Apples

You can use whole apples to make vinegar but this method takes about 7 months to complete.

10 apples

1 liter water

Procedure:

1. Wash the apple and cut it into quarters. Leave it in a plate covered with cheesecloth until it turns brown.
2. Place it in a glass bowl and add water. Cover the bowl with cheesecloth.
3. Place in a cool and dark place for 6 months.
4. You may notice that there is a grayish scum on the surface of the liquid. This is normal. Simply skim the scum off the top and strain the liquid into another bowl. Let it age for 6 weeks then transfer to a clean container.

Chapter 5: Apple Cider Vinegar Salad Dressing Recipes

Salad dressing is used to complement vegetables and fruits. It also encourages people to eat more whole produce. Apple cider vinegar has a subtle taste so it can be combined well with other ingredients.

Apple Cider Vinaigrette

¼ cup white vinegar
2 tbsp agave syrup
¼ tsp black pepper
1 ½ tbsp minced shallots
¼ cup apple cider vinegar
1 tbsp Dijon mustard
¼ tsp salt
½ cup canola oil

Makes 2/3 cup

Mix the vinegar, Dijon mustard, salt, agave syrup and black pepper in a bowl. Whisk the ingredients to combine. Add the oil slowly then whisk the mixture again. Add the shallots and serve.

Creamy Caesar Dressing

2 tsp apple cider vinegar
½ tsp mustard
2 garlic clove, crushed
2 tbsp Parmesan cheese
1 egg yolk, room temperature
1/3 cup olive oil
1 tbsp fresh lemon juice
2 tsp Worcestershire
Salt, spices and pepper to taste

Makes 1 cup

Whisk the egg in a bowl. Add the remaining ingredients then whisk again until combined. Make sure that the mixture is creamy. If the ingredients are not incorporated well, your egg might have been too cold.

Italian Zest

1 tsp Dijon mustard
½ tsp onion powder
½ tsp thyme
½ tsp oregano
½ tsp basil
3 tbsp apple cider vinegar
¼ cup olive oil
2 garlic cloves
Salt and pepper to taste

Makes 2/3 cup

Combine all of the ingredients in a bowl then stir to combine.

Greek Dressing

2 tbsp apple cider vinegar
½ tsp marjoram
½ tsp oregano
1 garlic clove, crushed
½ cup olive oil
1 tsp Dijon mustard
Salt and pepper to taste
½ tsp lemon juice

Makes 2/3 cup

Place all of the ingredients in a small jar. Shake vigorously to combine. Pour then serve.

Sweet Asian Vinaigrette

3 tbsp apple cider vinegar
2 tsp honey
Spices to taste
1/3 cup olive oil

2 tsp coconut amino
Pinch of ginger powder

Makes 2/3 cup

Combine ingredients in a blender. Process it until smooth.

Raspberry and Apple Cider Vinegar

¼ cup olive oil
2 tsp honey
½ cup apple cider vinegar
¼ cup raspberries

Blend the ingredients until smooth. Serve immediately.

French Dressing

1 tbsp tomato paste
¼ cup apple cider vinegar
½ tsp onion powder
1 squirt mustard
1/3 cup olive oil
1 tbsp honey

Makes 1 cup

Combine ingredients in a bowl or blender. Whisk until smooth. Pour in a bowl and serve.

Creamy Apple Cider Dressing

1 lemon, juiced
2 tbsp apple cider vinegar
2 tbsp fresh dill, chopped
¼ cup extra virgin olive oil
Salt and pepper to taste
3 tbsp honey
½ tsp cardamom
2 tsp Dijon mustard
3 tbsp cream

Makes 2/3 cup

Combine the lemon juice, dill, vinegar, honey and mustard in a bowl. Whisk to combine. Slowly add the oil. Whisk until fully incorporated. Add the cream and season with salt and pepper.

Chapter 6: Apple Cider Vinegar Drink Recipes

Drinking apple cider vinegar does not have to taste bland or boring. Try these apple cider vinegar drink recipes.

Lemon water and apple cider vinegar

1 glass of water
1 tbsp lemon juice
1 pinch of cayenne pepper
1 tbsp apple cider vinegar
½ tsp ground cinnamon

Makes 1 glass

Combine all of the ingredients in you glass of water. Stir to combine then serve.

Cranberry Detox Drink

¼ cup pure cranberry juice
1 tbsp lemon juice
Honey to taste
1 tbsp apple cider vinegar
Water

Makes 2 glasses

Add the ingredients in a large pitcher. You can adjust the water content as you prefer.

Green tea apple cider vinegar

1 cup green tea
Honey to taste
1 tbsp apple cider vinegar

Makes 1 cup

Boil water and pour in a cup. Seep the green tea and wait for several minutes. Let it cool before adding the apple cider vinegar.

Zingy cocktail

2 tbsp apple cider vinegar
1 ½ cups water
2 tbsp cranberry juice
2 tsp maple syrup

Makes 1 tall glass

Combine the ingredients in a tall glass then stir. Chill and serve.

Sweet Blaster

2 tbsp apple cider vinegar
2 tsp black strap molasses
1 ½ cups water

Makes 1 tall glass

This is a great morning drink. Combine all of the ingredients in a tall glass of water.

Tomato Cider Slinger

2 tbsp apple cider vinegar
1 ½ cups fresh or canned tomato juice
Pinch of salt

Makes 1 tall glass

Combine ingredients in a glass. Stir then serve.

Pink Juice

2 tsp raw honey
1 ½ cups grapefruit juice
2 tbsp apple cider vinegar

Makes 1 tall glass

Stir the ingredients in a glass. The juice is great to consume before your meals.

The Shot

1 tbsp apple juice
1 tbsp apple cider vinegar

Combine the ingredients in a shot glass. Just drink it straight up. It is better if you hold your breath and wash it down with chaser afterwards.

Chapter 7: Simple Apple Cider Vinegar Meal Recipes

Grilled Apple Cider Vinegar Chicken

1/3 cup light brown sugar
Fresh black pepper
¾ cup salt
5 lb chicken, cut into 8 pieces
For the basting liquid:
¼ cup canola oil
1 tbsp hot sauce
½ cup apple cider vinegar
2 tbsp Worcestershire sauce

Makes 8 servings

Prepare the brine and chicken. Mix the brown sugar, salt and 1 gallon of water in a container. Stir until it is dissolved. Add the chicken and refrigerate for 4 hours. Prepare the grill.

Make the basting liquid by whisking the water, oil, sauce and vinegar in a large bowl. Set this aside. Drain the chicken and season with pepper. Place on the grill. Cook for 2-3 minutes on each side. Turn it several times. Coat it with the basting liquid. Remove it from the grill and transfer to plate.

Veal Shanks with Apple Cider Vinegar

8 veal shins, center cut
5 tbsp butter
2 Granny Smith apples, peeled, cored and sliced
½ cup calvados
1 cup chicken stock
3 tbsp tarragon, minced
Salt to taste
4 cups all-purpose flour, seasoned
7 shallots, minced
2 ½ cups apple cider vinegar
½ cup heavy cream

½ cup currants

Makes 8 servings

Set the oven at 350 degrees. Coat the veal shanks with the flour. Cook the veal in the pan over high heat. Cook for 10 minutes then lower the temperature. Continue to cook for another 5 minutes. Watch it carefully so that it does not burn.

Cook the shallots and apples in the same pan. Once it is soft, add the vinegar and calvados. Let the mixture boil until the liquid is reduced in half. Add the chicken broth and boil the mixture.

Place the pan in the oven. Cover with foil then bake for 30-40 minutes until tender. Skim the fat from the mixture. Add the tarragon and cream. Cook for 5 minutes. Season it with salt and currants.

Glazed salmon with braised fennel

Braised fennel:
4 fennel bulbs, cut into wedges
1 cup apple cider
2 thyme sprigs
¼ cup parsley leaves, chopped
4 tbsp butter
3 tbsp sugar
1 cup chicken stock
Salt and pepper
For the glaze:
1 tsp cayenne pepper
Grape seed oil
Salt and pepper to taste
1 cup apple cider vinegar
3 tbsp brown sugar
8 oz boneless and skinless salmon fillet

Makes 4 servings

Set the oven at 425 degrees Fahrenheit. Make the braised fennel. Melt the butter in your Dutch oven. Add the sugar and fennel. Cook for 4 minutes until it is tender. Add the thyme, stock and cider vinegar. Cook until the liquid is reduced. Adjust the seasoning with salt and pepper. Add the parsley. Stir well to combine. Remove the mixture from the heat.

Make the glaze. Combine the cayenne, sugar and apple cider vinegar and heat until only one half cup of the liquid remains. Set this aside. Season the salmon fillet with salt and pepper. Add oil to your frying pan. Cook the fillet for 4 minutes at each side. Remove from the heat and spoon the glaze on top. Remove the mixture from the oven and serve with the braised fennel.

Brussels Sprouts with Bacon
3 lb medium Brussels sprouts
8 thick bacon slices
½ tsp salt
2 tbsp olive oil
3 tbsp apple cider vinegar
Black pepper to taste

Makes 3-4 servings

Boil a large pot of water and add the salt. Cut the end of the Brussels sprouts. Make sure that you keep the core intact. Remove the outer leaves. Slice the core in two. Cook the Brussels in the water for 5-7 minutes. Drain and let it cool for 10 minutes.

Add the oil in a pan. Cook the bacon in medium heat until crispy. Remove and place on top of the paper towel to drain excess fat. Add the Brussels sprouts and stir occasionally until it is crispy. Add the salt, pepper, bacon and apple cider vinegar.

Sweet potato with maple glazed pecans

3 ¼ lb sweet potatoes, washed and cut into chunks

½ tsp salt
Juice of 1 orange
2 tbsp canola oil
¼ tsp fresh ground black pepper
3 tbsp maple syrup
For the pecans:
2 tbsp pure maple syrup
1 tsp minced rosemary leaves
2 cups pecans
1 tbsp apple cider vinegar
¼ salt and pepper

Makes 4-6 servings

Set the oven at 400 degrees. Add the sweet potatoes in a shallow dish. Season it with salt, pepper and oil. Stir everything together until it is tender. This usually takes about 20 minutes. Stir the orange juice and maple syrup. Pour into the sweet potato mixture. Roast until the sweet potatoes are tender.

Prepare the pecans. Line the baking sheet with parchment paper. Combine the syrup, pecans, rosemary, salt, pepper and apple cider vinegar in a bowl. Toss the ingredients to combine. Spread in the baking pan. Bake for 15 minutes then let it cool. Use a fork to mash the sweet potatoes in the bowl. Spread it on the pan. Sprinkle the chopped pecans on top of the mixture before serving.

Vegan Wild Rice Stuffed Butternut Squash

3 tbsp apple cider vinegar
4 tbsp olive oil
1 small onion, chopped
½ tsp curry powder
1/ tsp cayenne pepper
1 cup loosely packed parsley leaves, chopped
¼ cup walnuts, coarsely chopped
2 medium butternut squash

2 tbsp maple syrup
Salt and pepper to taste
½ cup wild rice
½ tsp ground cinnamon
3 tbsp dried unsweetened cherries
1 tbsp fresh sage, chopped

Makes 4 servings

Place the oven rack in the middle of the oven. Set it at 400
degrees. Cut the squash lengthwise and remove the seeds. Arrange
it in the baking sheet with the flesh side up. Whisk the vinegar, oil
and maple syrup. Brush the liquid on the squash halves. Sprinkle
with salt and pepper. Coat the skin side of the butternut squash.
Sprinkle with salt and pepper. Roast for 40 minutes. Let it cool
then scoop the flesh.

Pour oil in a medium sized saucepan. Add the onions and cook for
3-5 minutes until it is soft and brown. Add the cayenne, cinnamon,
salt, spices, curry and rice. Add the water and simmer. Continue to
cook until most of the liquid is absorbed. Different brands of wild
rice may need more water. Scoop then add it to the butternut
mixture. Add the parsley, sage, salt, cherries and maple oil. Stuff
the filling into the butternut squash. Drizzle with the oil and bake
for 30 minutes or until it is warm. Sprinkle the parsley and
walnuts. Serve it while it is still warm.

German Potato Salad

2 lb white potatoes cut in half
Extra virgin olive oil
1 onion, diced
¼ cup apple cider vinegar
Salt to taste
8 bacon slices
½ cup chicken stock
1 bunch chives

Makes 3-4 servings

Place the potatoes in a medium pan. Add water and season it with salt. Boil and simmer until the potatoes are tender. Drain the liquid. Coat the pan with olive oil. Add the bacon in the pan and cook until it is crispy. Add the onions and cook until it is soft and fragrant. This usually takes about 8 minutes. Add the potatoes and cook until most of the liquid is absorbed. Adjust the seasoning if needed. Add the chives and serve at room temperature.

Black Beans and Rice

¼ cup olive oil
2 green bell peppers, chopped
4 bay leaves
2 cups long grain white rice
14 oz diced tomatoes
½ cup apple cider vinegar
2 onions, finely chopped
3 garlic cloves, chopped
1 tbsp ground cumin
14 oz black beans, drained and rinsed
2 cups water
 Salt and pepper to taste

Makes 4 servings

Place the pot over medium heat then add the oil. Cook the onions, bay leaf, cumin, garlic and pepper. Stir and cook until it is tender and fragrant. Add the black beans, water, vinegar, salt and tomatoes. Boil and cook for 30 minutes at high heat. Serve with the rice.

Broccoli Cole Slaw

3 bag ramen noodles

¼ cup slivered almonds
¼ cup sunflower seeds
Butter
24 oz broccoli cole slaw
Green onions for garnish
For the dressing:
¼ cup honey
Salt and pepper to taste
¾ cup olive oil
2/3 cup apple cider vinegar

Makes 2-3 servings

Place the ramen noodles in a sealable bag. Crush it using a rolling pin. Pour in a large bowl then add the almonds. Cook it in a pan over medium heat. Whisk all of the dressing ingredients in a bowl. Combine the broccoli, almonds and sunflower seeds in a separate bowl. Pour the dressing and stir to coat. Garnish with the green onions.

Apple Cider Pork Tenderloin

2 lbs pork tenderloin, cut crosswise
Salt and pepper to taste
1/2 cup apple cider vinegar
Olive oil
1 ½ cups apple cider
¼ cup maple syrup

Makes 4 servings

Set the oven at 500 degrees. Coat the pork with oil and season with salt and pepper. Heat the pan. Cook the pork for 4 minutes on each side. Transfer it to the baking sheet. Bake for 15 minutes.

Combine the cider and vinegar in a pan. Cook until the liquid is reduced. Add the maple syrup. Spoon the sauce over the pork. Let it cool then slice thinly. Serve with extra sauce.

Chapter 8: Other Helpful Uses For Apple Cider Vinegar

Apple cider vinegar can be used for other things besides adding it to your salads and drinks. Here are some ways on how you can incorporate apple cider vinegar into your daily regimen.

Home Use

Apple cider vinegar can be used as a natural disinfectant. It can also be used for your gardens and even pets.

- Nontoxic all-purpose cleaner

Commercial sprays and solution may be effective in removing tough stains but it also contains chemicals that can be dangerous to your health. Apple cider vinegar is also a natural disinfectant. People have been using apple cider vinegar for centuries to keep their houses clean and odor-free. Simply combine the apple cider vinegar with water. Pour it into a spray bottle and use it just like any cleansing spray.

- Remove unwanted odor

Keep you rooms smelling clean and fresh with apple cider vinegar. It is effective against cigarette smoke and unwanted bathroom odor. Pour the apple cider vinegar in a bowl and leave it in the room. Leave it there until the smell vanishes.

- Garden helper

You can boost the vitality of your garden using apple cider vinegar, because you can use it as a fertilizer. It is especially effective on plants that love acid such as azalea and blueberry bushes. Apple cider vinegar is also effective in preventing weeds from damaging your plants. Dilute 10 oz of apple cider vinegar with 10 gallons of water.

- Keep your pet flea free

One of the common problems when it comes to pets is flea infestation. Dilute the apple cider with water and work it into their fur and skin. Let it stay for 20 minutes then rinse it off.

Face and Body Use

People who are looking for natural, economical and effective beauty treatments will delight in using apple cider vinegar. It provides a lot of benefits and can be used in different ways.

- Gets rid of dandruff

Apple cider vinegar can change your skin's pH level to stop yeast growth and help prevent dandruff. The vinegar can also get rid of irritation, greasiness and oil. Mix one tablespoon of the vinegar in a glass of water and rinse your hair in the shower. For severe dandruff cases, you can dilute ¼ cup of vinegar with ¼ cup of water. Massage it in your scalp and leave it for an hour before you rinse it off.

- Improve complexion

Apple cider can kill bacteria in the surface of the skin and reduce acne. You can use it as a toner or as a spot treatment for your blemishes. Regularly using apple cider vinegar can also help unclog pores to keep you skin fresh and clean.

- Alternative to commercial deodorant

Apple cider vinegar can help control body odor. Pour it in a cotton ball and apply on your under arm. The smell of vinegar evaporates quickly so you do not have to worry about smelling like a salad all day.

- Relive burnt skin and fade bruises

Diluted apple cider vinegar can sooth burnt skin and helps it heal faster. Apple cider vinegar has anti-inflammatory properties that can fade bruises faster.

- Get rid of warts

Warts can develop on anyone. You can use apple cider vinegar to remove the warts gently. Douse the cotton ball in the vinegar then secure it in your warts. Leave overnight.

- Whiten teeth and freshens breath

Apple cider vinegar can whiten your teeth especially if you combine it with baking soda. You can also use it as a mouthwash to remove germs and bacteria in the mouth. Simply gargle with the apple cider vinegar for a minute then spit it out.

- Foot deodorizer

Keep your feet fresh by rubbing apple cider vinegar on your feet. It can kill bacteria that causes odor. Make sure that you rub the solution in between your toes.

- Aftershave

Reduce the risk of ingrown hair and infection by applying apple cider vinegar on your freshly shaven skin. Make sure that you dilute it in water. The smell of vinegar will evaporate quickly.

Health and Wellness

One of the reasons why apple cider is very popular is because of its health benefits.

- Sooth your upset stomach

Your stomach is susceptible to many pains and diseases. It is exposed to millions of bacteria every day because of the food that you consume. Drinking apple cider vinegar with water can help resolve the problem. It has antibacterial and antiviral properties that can sooth you stomach.

- Relive muscle soreness

Apple cider vinegar contains acetic acid that can sooth aching muscles when applied topically. Try to use it instead of regular lotion.

- Helps relive diabetes

If you were diagnosed with diabetes, you will be glad to know that apple cider vinegar can help you with your ailment. Ingesting apple cider can help keep your blood sugar stable. It can also improve insulin sensitivity and prevent type 2 diabetes.

- Relive sore throat

Apple cider can relive sore throat before it becomes more serious. Just mix ¼ cup of apple cider vinegar with warm water and gargle. This creates an acidic environment in your throat, which can kill germs in your throat. You can also create a tonic by mixing apple cider vinegar, pepper and honey.

- Clear your sinus

Having a stuffed nose can be exhausting. Clear your sinuses using apple cider vinegar and water. This can help prevent bacteria from growing in your sinus. The potassium content of the apple cider mixture can thin out the mucus in your nose.

- Helps you feel more energized

Take a break from energy drinks that are full of sugar. If you are filling a little down, you can make a natural booster by combining apple cider vinegar with juice or water.

- Stop itch

Apple cider vinegar can help with bug bites, jellyfish stings and poison ivy. Just apply the mixture in your skin and let the apple cider take effect.

Conclusion

Thank you again for purchasing this book on apple cider vinegar!

I am extremely excited to pass this information along to you, and I am so happy that you now have read and can hopefully implement these strategies going forward.

I hope this book was able to help you understand the benefits of apple cider and how to use it in home remedies and recipes.

The next step is to get started using this information and to hopefully live a happy and healthy life!

Please don't be someone who just reads this information and doesn't apply it, the strategies in this book will only benefit you if you use them!

If you know of anyone else that could benefit from the information presented here please inform them of this book.

Finally, if you enjoyed this book and feel it has added value to your life in any way, please take the time to share your thoughts and post a review on Amazon. It'd be greatly appreciated!

Thank you and good luck!

Preview Of:

Ultimate Get In Shape Guide!

<u>Weight Loss</u>

Metabolism Secrets, Diet Tricks, And HIIT High Intensity Interval Training For Fast Fat Loss And To Build Muscle Fast!

Introduction

I want to thank you and congratulate you for purchasing the book, *"Weight Loss!"*

This book contains proven steps and strategies on how to get in shape with HIIT and dieting.

Getting in shape is the combination of having the right knowledge, setting realistic goals and having the motivation to do it.

One aspect of a healthy lifestyle is committing to a healthy diet. Different types of diet can work for different people and the main key is to find one that fits your lifestyle. You also have to remember to get enough nutrients to make sure that you are performing at your maximum capacity.

You cannot get in shape without exercising. Humans are genetically designed to be active. HIIT exercise is an efficient and quick workout which you can do almost anywhere. You can also add other physical activities that you like.

This book also contains many tips on how you can stay motivated to reach your goal. Everyone gets discouraged at times but those who succeed always find a way to conquer challenges and achieve better results.

Thanks again for purchasing this book, I hope you enjoy it!

Chapter 1: The Main Reason Most People Never Get In Shape

Committing to a healthy lifestyle can be difficult most especially for people who have never considered it before. It is easy to find a reason to skip workouts and keep on eating junk food all the time.

Here are the top reasons why most people never get in shape:

Busy schedule

People who have a rigid work schedule may reason that they cannot find enough time to exercise. However, unless you work for 16 hours a day seven days in a week, most people can squeeze in 30 minutes of exercise a day. You can even take few minutes break from work every few hours to walk or stretch in place.

If you do not have enough time, you can break up your workout routine into shorter sessions. Remember that having a little bit of workout is better than none at all. Also, people who are really committed to healthy lifestyle find time to work out no matter their work schedule.

Low energy

After a day's work, some prefer to relax at home and watch TV instead of working out. Exercise actually gives people more energy and increases their stamina. Working out triggers the production of endorphin which can make you feel good and also improves better blood circulation.

You can also exercise first thing in the morning before you find excuse to skip it later. Again, you don't have to do a vigorous workout. You can simply jog for half an hour whenever you feel best.

Family responsibilities

Taking care of your children can take a toll on your schedule but it is not an excuse to stop working out. Taking your children in the park can be both fun and functional. You can spend time playing with them and exercise at the same time. There are a lot of activities you can enjoy with your kids like running or riding a bike around the neighborhood. Also, you will be setting a good example for your children if they see their parents living a healthy and active lifestyle.

Boring exercise

The best way to combat boredom is to find an activity that you enjoy. There are a lot of exercises that can fit any preference and personality. You should also switch up your routine every few months to avoid losing motivation. You can also enlist some friends or join a group to have more motivation.

Unhealthy diet

A person can commit to an exercise routine but they won't be able to get in shape if they do not change their unhealthy diet. Although not all diets can suit everybody, there is always a diet principle that can fit your lifestyle. All you have to do is to research and find it. Eating a balanced diet from carbohydrates, protein and fat is a good start. Remember that a healthy lifestyle is composed of healthy eating and enough exercise.

Tried before

Most people have tried to get in shape once or twice in their life. Some people succeed in their fitness goal while others fail. Those who fail might lose their motivation and decide not to try again. Set smaller and realistic goals next time. This way when you succeed in your goal, you are more motivated to accomplish another one.

Thanks for Previewing My Exciting Book Entitled:

"Weight Loss: Metabolism Secrets, Diet Tricks, And HIIT High Intensity Interval Training For Fast Fat Loss And To Build Muscle Fast!"

To purchase this book, simply go to the Amazon Kindle store and simply search:

"WEIGHT LOSS"

Then just scroll down until you see my book. You will know it is mine because you will see my name "Sarah Brooks" underneath the title.

Alternatively, you can visit my author page on Amazon to see this book and other work I have done. Thanks so much, and please don't forget your free bonuses

DON'T LEAVE YET! - CHECK OUT YOUR FREE BONUSES BELOW!

Free Bonus Offer: Get Free Access To The www.LiveFitVIP.com VIP News-letter!

Once you enter your email address you will immediately get free access to this awesome newsletter!

But wait, right now if you join now for free you will also get free access to the "The 7 Keys To Body Transformation" free EBook!

To claim both your FREE VIP NEWSLETTER MEMBERSHIP and your FREE BONUS EBook on THE 7 KEYS TO BODY TRANSFORMATION!

Just Go To:

www.liveFitVIP.com